Breaking the Insulin Resistance Cycle:

Effective Management and Reversal Strategies

By

Christopher M. McIntosh

Breaking the Insulin Resistance Cycle:

Effective Management and Reversal Strategies with Proven Techniques for Regulating Blood Sugar Levels, Losing Weight, and Restoring Metabolic Health.

Breaking the Insulin Resistance Cycle

Table of Content

Breaking the Insulin Resistance Cycle

Introduction

Millions of people worldwide are impacted by the growing epidemic of insulin resistance. The disorder causes the body to become less receptive to the hormone insulin, which raises blood glucose levels. Type 2 diabetes, heart disease, and other major health consequences may potentially result from this

Despite its prevalence, there is hope for those suffering from insulin resistance. It is feasible to reverse insulin resistance and stop the onset of more serious health problems with correct management and lifestyle adjustments.

The goal of this book is to give readers a thorough manual for controlling insulin resistance and reaching optimum health. Together with the most recent findings and treatment options, we will examine the causes, signs, and effects of insulin resistance. We will go over all the methods and instruments required to increase insulin sensitivity and reverse insulin resistance, from dietary adjustments and exercise regimens to medications and supplements.

This book will provide you with the information and tools you need to control your health and reclaim your life, whether you have insulin resistance for the first time or have been dealing with it for some time. So let's get started on the path to a healthier, happier you!

Chapter 1

Understanding Insulin and Insulin Resistance

The hormone insulin is essential for controlling the body's metabolism. When blood glucose (sugar) levels rise, it is created by the pancreatic beta cells and delivered into the bloodstream.

Breaking the Insulin Resistance Cycle

Insulin affects cells all over the body once it enters the bloodstream, but it has a particular impact on adipose (fat) tissue, the liver, and muscles. By boosting glucose uptake into cells and storage as glycogen or fat, it lowers blood glucose levels as one of its main goals.

Insulin encourages the liver to turn extra glucose into glycogen, which can be kept for future use. Insulin promotes the uptake of glucose, which can be used as energy during physical activity, in muscle cells. Insulin works in adipose tissue.

The body uses insulin for a number of other essential purposes, such as:

Preventing the release of glucose from the liver and the breakdown of glycogen

Encouraging the synthesis of proteins and the development and repair of tissues

Improving the absorption of amino acids, the protein building blocks, into cells.

Preventing the breakdown of fat reserves and encouraging fat storage

In a nutshell, insulin controls several aspects of the body's metabolism, including the intake and storage of glucose, protein synthesis, and the storage and breakdown of fat. The maintenance of normal blood sugar levels and general health and well-being depend on insulin.

What exactly is insulin, and why is it important?

The pancreas' beta cells create the hormone insulin. Its main function is to control the blood's level of glucose

Breaking the Insulin Resistance Cycle

(sugar). The body's metabolism depends on insulin, which is also necessary for general health and well-being.

The body converts the food we eat, mainly carbs, into glucose, which is then absorbed into the bloodstream. The pancreas releases insulin as blood glucose levels rise, telling cells all over the body to either take up glucose and use it as energy right away or store it for later.

The fact that insulin helps to regulate blood glucose levels and prevents them from rising too high (hyperglycemia) or falling too low (hypoglycemia), over time, excessive blood glucose levels can harm organs, nerves, and blood vessels. Diabetes, heart disease, renal damage, and other health issues might result from this. Shaking, confusion and fainting are symptoms that can result from low blood sugar levels.

In addition to these vital functions, insulin also aids in tissue growth and repair and controls how fat and protein are broken down and stored in the body. Type 2 diabetes and other metabolic diseases, including insulin resistance, happen when the body's cells stop responding to insulin.

Breaking the Insulin Resistance Cycle

Insulin is an essential hormone that controls blood glucose levels and is crucial for maintaining general health and avoiding a number of diseases.

Insulin and carbohydrates differ from one another

We consume two types of carbohydrates: refined and complex. Whole grains, vegetables, fruits in their full form, nuts, and legumes are a few examples of complex carbohydrates. Particularly legumes can assist with naturally reversing insulin resistance. White rice, white flour, and sugar are a few examples of refined carbohydrates. Natural insulin resistance reversal occurs in legumes. Once ingested, all carbs are converted to sugar. Certain things degrade more slowly than others. Low-glycemic carbs, which include legumes, apples, cherries, and above-ground vegetables, are those that digest slowly. Some carbs degrade more quickly. Excessive consumption of high glycemic index carbohydrates causes the most sugar storage in the body. Excessive intake of all carbohydrates, especially the high-glycemic type, is the primary culprit in the development of insulin resistance. These are called high glycemic carbohydrates. Examples are wheat, rice, tubers, vegetables (potatoes), watermelon, and bananas. Once converted to sugar inside the body, carbohydrates encourage the pancreas to release more insulin. As the body tries to remove the excess sugar from the blood and store it somewhere else, there is a commensurate rise in blood sugar and an immediate rise in insulin every time there is a rise in sugar in the diet (such as after eating a large bowl of noodles). The body balances itself to maintain a steady blood sugar level, therefore this process happens automatically. Although sugar is a useful source of energy, it was never intended to be the main one. Sugar is intended to be used as a temporary emergency fuel, such as when evading danger. Certainly, our brains will use sugar as fuel, but it doesn't have to. It can do very well by burning

ketones from fats. Fats and triglycerides can then be converted into sugar for emergency use. The body prefers using fat as an energy source.

Furthermore, the body can function just fine without simple, refined carbs as long as there is enough protein and fat to supply the calories needed for metabolic processes. Our bodies are made to use fats, not sugar, as fuel. In reality, since fat is the preferred energy source, excess sugar is stored as fat. The body has a large capacity for fat but a smaller capacity for sugar.

In terms of the body, sugar is a known poison if consumed in large quantities. The easiest way for the body to get rid of these extra sugars is by burning them. Glycogen is the

Breaking the Insulin Resistance Cycle

form that the body stores whatever it cannot burn. When that is full, it transforms into fat. The body will burn sugar before fat when you consume sugar. Bloodstream sugar will be consumed first, followed by glycogen, which is stored sugar. Our blood sugar levels rise rapidly. The body panics because it does not appreciate the surge. Immediately after receiving the signal, the pancreas releases insulin to help transport sugar from the bloodstream into the cell, decreasing blood sugar levels. This response is a backup since our bodies weren't designed to process large amounts of sugar quickly; rather, they should only seldom do so.

How does insulin resistance form and what does it entail?

Breaking the Insulin Resistance Cycle

A condition known as insulin resistance occurs when the body's cells stop responding to the effects of insulin. This means that for the same effect on blood glucose levels, the body needs more insulin. High blood glucose levels, a crucial aspect of type 2 diabetes, can eventually result from insulin resistance.

Insulin resistance and obesity, especially extra weight around the abdomen, are frequently

Breaking the Insulin Resistance Cycle

linked. Although the specific causes of insulin resistance are not fully known, it is believed that a complex interplay between genetic, environmental, and lifestyle variables is at play.

One theory is that excess body fat, particularly in the abdominal area, can release inflammatory chemicals that interfere with insulin signaling pathways in the body. This can cause the body's cells to become less responsive to insulin over time.

 Other risk factors for insulin resistance include:

Aging

Sedentary lifestyle

Poor diet, particularly a diet high in processed and sugary foods

Sleep deprivation

Chronic stress

Insulin resistance can emerge gradually over a long period of time and may not initially manifest any symptoms. High blood sugar levels can, however, eventually cause a number of health issues, such as kidney damage, nerve damage, visual issues, heart disease, and other issues. A variety of tests, including those that measure fasting glucose and insulin levels, glucose tolerance, and hemoglobin A1c, can be used to identify insulin resistance. It can be controlled with a mix of medication, such as insulin-sensitizing medications, and lifestyle adjustments, such as a nutritious diet and regular exercise. Type 2 diabetes and other associated health issues can be prevented by early detection and management of insulin resistance.

Risk factors for insulin resistance and type 2 diabetes

A significant risk factor for type 2 diabetes is insulin resistance, and both diseases share a number of other risk factors. The following are some of the major risk factors for type 2 diabetes and insulin resistance:

Obesity: Being overweight, especially around the waist, increases the risk of developing type 2 diabetes and insulin resistance.

Sedentary lifestyle: Lack of exercise and excessive sitting time can raise the risk of type 2 diabetes and insulin resistance.

Bad diet: Eating a lot of sugary, processed foods, refined carbohydrates, and unhealthy fats will make you more likely to develop insulin resistance and type 2 diabetes.

Family history: Type 2 diabetes and insulin resistance

are illnesses that are more likely to run in families.

Age: As people age, their chance of developing type 2 diabetes and insulin resistance rises.

Ethnicity: Type 2 diabetes and insulin resistance are more common in some groups of people, including African Americans, Hispanic/Latino Americans, and Native Americans.

Gestational diabetes: Women who have experienced gestational diabetes during pregnancy are more likely to go on to have type 2 diabetes and insulin resistance in the future.

Polycystic ovarian syndrome (PCOS): PCOS is a hormonal disease that puts women at a higher risk of developing insulin resistance and type 2 diabetes.

Breaking the Insulin Resistance Cycle

Persistent sleep loss or poor quality sleep can raise the risk of insulin resistance and type 2 diabetes.

It's crucial to remember that having one or more of these risk factors does not guarantee that you will develop type 2 diabetes or insulin resistance. Several risk factors, however, can increase your overall risk. Changing your lifestyle to include good eating, regular exercise, maintaining a healthy weight, and stress management will help to lower your chance of acquiring these disorders.

Chapter 2

Diagnosis and Monitoring of Insulin Resistance

How is insulin resistance diagnosed?

Usually, a combination of blood testing and physical examinations is used to detect insulin resistance. The following are the most typical tests used to identify insulin resistance:

Haemoglobin A1c (HbA1c)

test: This test measures the average blood glucose level over the past two to three months. It helps establish whether treatment programs are effective by tracking blood glucose management over time.

Fasting plasma glucose (FPG)

test: This test measures the blood glucose level after an overnight fast. It is used to identify diabetes patients and track their blood glucose

levels.

Oral glucose tolerance test

(OGTT): This test involves

drinking a sugary drink and

measuring blood glucose

levels at various intervals. It is

used to identify diabetics and

track their blood glucose

levels.

Random plasma glucose test:

Regardless of when the person

last had food, this test gauges

blood glucose levels at any

given moment. It is used to identify diabetes patients and track their blood glucose levels.

Fructosamine test: This test measures the average blood glucose level over the past two to three weeks. It is utilized to check on the management of blood glucose in diabetics.

Insulin level test: This examination determines the amount of insulin present in the body. It is used to track insulin resistance and assess how well insulin resistance therapies are working.

In addition to these tests, other markers of diabetes and insulin resistance, such as blood pressure and cholesterol levels, may also be monitored to help manage the condition. A physical exam and medical history review may also be used to diagnose insulin resistance. Doctors may ask questions about diet, exercise habits, family history of diabetes or other related health conditions, and other lifestyle factors that may contribute to insulin resistance.

It's crucial to remember that insulin resistance frequently appears gradually over time and may not initially manifest any symptoms. Insulin resistance, however, can eventually result in type 2 diabetes and excessive blood sugar levels if it is not managed. It's crucial to identify and treat insulin resistance early on if you want to avoid more significant health issues.

When choosing the tests that are best for monitoring insulin resistance and diabetes, it's essential to consult a healthcare professional. The treatment strategy and the individual's specific needs will determine how frequently tests are administered. To guarantee that blood glucose levels are correctly maintained and to stop the emergence of linked health issues, regular monitoring is important.

Understanding blood sugar levels and glycemic control

The amount of glucose in the blood is measured by blood sugar readings. The main source of energy for the body is glucose, which is obtained from the food we eat.

Breaking the Insulin Resistance Cycle

Following a meal, the body converts carbs into glucose, which travels through the blood and provides energy to the body's cells.

The ability of the body to maintain blood glucose levels within a normal range is referred to as glycemic control. Because high or low blood glucose levels can result in a variety of health issues, maintaining good blood sugar levels is crucial for general health and well-being.

For the majority of people, the normal range for blood glucose levels is between 70 and 140 mg/dL (milligrams per deciliter). However, the normal range can vary depending on a person's age, health status, and other factors.

Hyperglycemia, often known as high blood sugar, can occur when the body is unable to adequately make or utilize insulin. Anyone with type 2 diabetes or insulin resistance may experience these. Increased thirst, frequent urination, impaired vision, lethargy, and sluggish wound healing are all signs of elevated blood sugar levels. When blood glucose levels go too low, hypoglycemia, or low blood sugar, can happen. This may be brought on by specific drugs like insulin or oral diabetic treatments, as well as other things like intense activity, drinking too much alcohol, or not eating enough. Dizziness, shakiness, sweating, confusion, and in severe cases, loss of consciousness, are all signs of low blood sugar. In order to maintain appropriate blood glucose levels, one must combine good lifestyle choices with any necessary medical care. Eating a balanced diet full of whole grains, fruits, and vegetables; engaging in regular physical activity; and taking medications as directed by a healthcare professional are some methods for maintaining appropriate blood glucose levels. To find the best strategy for preserving healthy blood glucose levels and attaining optimal glycemic control, see a healthcare professional.

Chapter 3

Lifestyle Strategies for Managing Insulin Resistance

Diet and nutrition recommendations for insulin resistance and diabetes

Food and nutrition play a significant role in managing diabetes and insulin resistance. Choosing nutritious food choices can enhance overall health and help control blood sugar levels. Here are a few food suggestions for diabetes and insulin resistance:

Putting whole foods first: A diet high in whole foods will help control blood sugar levels and enhance general health. These foods include fruits, vegetables, whole grains, lean proteins, and healthy fats. Because they frequently include a lot of refined carbs, added sugars, and harmful fats, processed and packaged foods should be avoided.

Reduce your intake of carbs because they cause your blood sugar levels to surge when they are broken down into glucose. Consuming fewer carbohydrates can help control blood sugar levels. Simple carbohydrates like refined sweets and processed foods should be avoided in favor of complex carbs like whole grains, legumes, and non-starchy vegetables.

Observe serving sizes: Even eating nutritious foods in excess might raise blood glucose levels. Controlling one's intake is crucial for maintaining healthy blood sugar levels.

Choose wholesome fats: Although fats are a necessary component of the diet, some fats are better for you than others. Olive oil, nuts, seeds, fish, and other foods high in mono- and polyunsaturated fatty acids have been shown to increase insulin sensitivity and reduce the risk of heart disease.

Limit saturated and trans-fats: Saturated and trans-fats can increase insulin resistance and contribute to the development of heart disease. These fats can be found in processed foods, full-fat dairy products, fatty meats, and other foods.

Eliminate added sugars from your diet: Added sugars are a key cause of insulin resistance and high blood sugar. Avoid drinking sugary beverages and eating candies and other sweets.

Select meals high in fiber since they can help control blood sugar levels and enhance general health. Fruits, vegetables, whole grains, and legumes are among the foods that are good providers of fiber.

As stated earlier on, in making healthy dietary choices, it's important to work with a healthcare provider to determine the best approach to managing insulin resistance and diabetes. Medical treatment, including medications and insulin therapy, may also be necessary to achieve optimal blood glucose control.

Exercise and physical activity for managing insulin resistance and diabetes

Exercise and regular physical activity are crucial for treating insulin resistance and diabetes. Exercise can help improve insulin sensitivity, regulate blood glucose levels, and lower the risk of cardiovascular disease.

Here are some suggestions for controlling insulin resistance

Breaking the Insulin Resistance Cycle

and diabetes through exercise and physical activity:

For at least 150 minutes of weekly moderate-intensity aerobic activity, aim for 30 minutes of exercise, five days a week. This category of exercise includes brisk walking, dancing, swimming, and cycling.

Including workouts for strength training in your routine: Exercises for strength training can increase muscle mass, which can enhance insulin sensitivity. Weightlifting, resistance band exercises, and bodyweight workouts like pushups and squats are a few examples of strength training exercises.

Be physically active throughout the day: It's crucial to be physically active throughout the day in addition to scheduled exercise. This can involve walking instead of driving for small distances, using the stairs instead of the elevator, or taking a quick walk after meals.

Monitor blood glucose levels before and after exercise: Exercise can cause changes in blood glucose levels, so it's crucial to check levels before and after to prevent hypoglycemia or hyperglycemia.

Think about collaborating with a medical professional or an expert in exercise: Working with a healthcare professional or exercise specialist to create a personalized fitness regimen that is safe and suitable for your requirements and medical history may be beneficial.

In addition to its physical advantages, exercise can also aid with stress reduction and mood enhancement, both of which are advantageous for general health and well-being. To find the best strategy for controlling insulin resistance and diabetes, it's crucial to discuss an exercise plan with a healthcare professional, just like with any lifestyle adjustment.

Management of stress and sleep for diabetes and insulin resistance

A key part of controlling insulin resistance and diabetes is getting enough sleep and managing your stress. High-stress levels and poor sleep quality can both lead to insulin resistance and high blood sugar levels. Here are some suggestions for controlling stress and sleep for treating diabetes and insulin resistance:

Strive for 7-8 hours of sleep each night: Obtaining enough sleep is essential for controlling blood sugar levels and lowering the chance of developing insulin resistance. Sleep quality can be enhanced by developing a reliable sleep schedule and a relaxing sleeping environment.

Reduce stress: Elevated blood sugar levels and insulin resistance can both be influenced by high amounts of stress. Stress levels can be lowered by partaking in stress-relieving activities like yoga, meditation, or deep breathing techniques.

Limit screen time before bed: Sleep patterns might be hampered by blue light exposure from electronics like smartphones and tablets. Reducing screen time before bed can enhance the quality of your sleep.

Avoid caffeine and alcohol before bedtime: As these chemicals might disrupt sleep cycles, it's crucial to avoid taking them before bed.

Work with a healthcare provider or mental health professional: It may be good to collaborate with a healthcare physician or mental health expert to create a plan that is specific to your requirements because managing stress and enhancing sleep quality can be difficult.

Enhancing sleep quality and lowering stress can have a good effect on general health and well-being and assist those with insulin resistance and diabetes in controlling blood glucose levels. It's crucial to discuss sleep and stress management techniques with a healthcare professional as with any lifestyle adjustment to find the best method for managing insulin resistance and diabetes.

Chapter 4

Medications and Insulin Therapy

Overview of medications used to manage insulin resistance and diabetes

There are several classes of medications used to manage insulin resistance and diabetes, including:

Metformin: One drug that is frequently used to treat type 2 diabetes is metformin. It functions by lowering liver glucose production and raising insulin sensitivity.

Sulfonylureas: Sulfonylureas are a group of drugs that encourage the pancreas to secrete more insulin. They frequently work better when combined with metformin to regulate blood sugar.

DPP-4 inhibitors: DPP-4 inhibitors are a more recent class of drugs that lower glucagon secretion and boost insulin secretion to assist control of blood sugar levels. To treat diabetes, they are frequently taken in addition to other drugs.

GLP-1 receptor agonists are a family of drugs that work similarly to the hormone GLP-1, which increases insulin secretion while decreasing glucagon secretion. To treat diabetes, they are frequently taken in addition to other drugs.

SGLT-2 inhibitors: SGLT-2 inhibitors are a class of drugs that increase glucose excretion in the urine by inhibiting the reabsorption of glucose by the kidneys. To treat diabetes, they are frequently taken in addition to other drugs.

Insulin: Insulin is a hormone produced by the pancreas that regulates blood glucose levels. Insulin therapy is necessary to manage the condition in people with type 1 diabetes and certain people with type 2 diabetes. Insulin can be administered via injection or an insulin pump.

How insulin therapy works and how to use insulin effectively

Breaking the Insulin Resistance Cycle

By replenishing the insulin that the body is unable to adequately manufacture or utilize, insulin treatment is used to manage diabetes. By imitating the body's natural insulin, insulin treatment helps to control blood glucose levels.

Insulin is injected into the subcutaneous tissue, or the fatty tissue beneath the skin, as part of insulin therapy. A syringe, an insulin pen, or an insulin pump can all be used to administer insulin. The insulin type and manner of administration will vary depending on the patient's medical history, blood glucose levels, and other health conditions.

To use insulin effectively, it's important to:

Obey the advice of the medical professional:

Following the healthcare provider's recommendations

for the kind of insulin, dose, and time of injections is crucial because insulin therapy is extremely customized.

Keep an eye on blood sugar levels: Regular blood glucose monitoring can be used to assess how well insulin therapy is working for you. A continuous glucose monitoring (CGM) system or a blood glucose meter can both be used to check blood sugar levels.

Know how to handle and store insulin: To prevent contamination, insulin must be handled carefully and kept in a cold, dry location. Understanding how to handle and store insulin is crucial for ensuring its efficacy.

Be mindful of any possible negative effects: Hypoglycemia (low blood glucose levels) and other side effects of insulin therapy are possible. It's crucial to understand potential side effects and know how to manage them.

Make lifestyle changes: Managing diabetes requires more than just insulin therapy; it also requires lifestyle changes including food and exercise. The amount of insulin required to control diabetes can be decreased by changing one's lifestyle, which can also assist improve one's insulin sensitivity.

Insulin therapy can be an effective way to manage diabetes, but it requires careful monitoring and management to be used effectively. Working closely with a healthcare provider and diabetes care team can help ensure that insulin therapy is used safely and effectively.

Understanding insulin dosing and injection techniques

Important components of insulin therapy for people with

diabetes include insulin dosage and injection technique. When giving insulin, it's important to keep the following things in mind:

Taking insulin: The dosage of insulin will change depending on a person's medical history, blood glucose levels, and other health conditions. Usually, medical professionals will give clear dose directions to follow.

Injection site: Usually, subcutaneous tissue in the abdomen, thighs or upper arms receives an injection of insulin. Alternating injection sites can ensure that insulin is regularly absorbed while preventing lipo-hypertrophy, or thickening or lumping of the skin.

Technique for administering an injection: Good injection technique can assist guarantee that insulin is effectively absorbed. Using a clean needle, creating a skin fold by pinching the skin, and injecting the insulin at a 90-degree angle are the steps in the injection procedure.

Time of injections: Depending on the type of insulin and the person's blood glucose levels, the timing of insulin injections will change. Long-acting insulin is often injected once or twice a day to provide basal insulin coverage, whereas rapid-acting insulin is typically administered before meals to cover the rise in blood glucose that happens after eating.

Devices for delivering insulin: A syringe, an insulin pen, or an insulin pump can all be used to administer insulin. The delivery strategy will be determined by a person's medical background, blood glucose levels, and other factors.

It's important to work closely with a healthcare provider and diabetes care team to ensure that insulin dosing and injection techniques are used effectively. Healthcare providers can provide specific instructions and guidance to help individuals use insulin safely and effectively.

Chapter 5

Advanced Strategies for Insulin Management and Possible Reversal

Use of insulin pumps and continuous glucose monitors (CGMs)

Insulin pumps and continuous glucose monitoring (CGM) devices are two cutting-edge technologies that can assist

Breaking the Insulin Resistance Cycle

people with diabetes in controlling their blood glucose levels.

To monitor the amount of glucose in the interstitial fluid (the liquid that surrounds the body's cells), CGM systems inject a tiny sensor beneath the skin. The receiver, which might be a handheld device, a smartphone, or a smart-watch, receives glucose level measurements from the sensor. Real-time glucose readings from CGM systems enable users to make quick changes to their insulin dosage, food, and exercise routine.

Insulin is continually delivered through a tiny, flexible tube that is put beneath the skin by small, battery-powered devices known as insulin pumps. The pump is set up to continuously supply an insulin flow that can be modified to meet a particular person's

Breaking the Insulin Resistance Cycle

demands. Moreover, the pump can be set up to provide bolus insulin dosages prior to meals or to lower high blood sugar levels.

Sensor-augmented pump therapy, which combines CGM and insulin pump therapy, can offer even more accurate glucose level control. CGM readings can be utilized to instantly change the settings on an insulin pump, enabling users to maintain ideal glucose control all through the day and night.

The use of CGM systems and insulin pumps can offer several benefits to individuals with diabetes, including:

Improved glucose control: CGM systems and insulin pumps can provide more precise glucose control, helping to prevent high and low blood glucose levels.

The risk of severe hypoglycemia is decreased because CGM devices can warn people when their blood sugar levels are low before symptoms appear.

Convenience boosted: Insulin pumps offer a constant infusion of the hormone, eliminating the need for repeated daily injections. Real-time glucose measurements from CGM devices eliminate the need for repeated finger-stick testing.

Better quality of life: CGM devices and insulin pumps can give users more flexibility in controlling their diabetes, making it simpler for them to incorporate diabetes management into daily activities.

CGM systems and insulin pumps are highly individualized and require close monitoring and management by a healthcare provider and diabetes care team. Working closely with a healthcare provider can help individuals determine if these advanced technologies are appropriate for their diabetes management needs.

Intermittent fasting and low-carbohydrate diets for insulin management

Low-carbohydrate diets and intermittent fasting are two nutritional strategies that may help some diabetics manage their insulin levels.

Cycling between fasting and eating phases is known as intermittent fasting. There are various forms of intermittent fasting, but time-restricted feeding, alternate-day fasting, and 5:2 fasting are the most popular.

With time-limited feeding, food intake is restricted to a certain time frame each day, such as an 8-hour window.

Breaking the Insulin Resistance Cycle

Alternating between days of regular eating and days of restricted calorie intake is known as alternate-day fasting. 5:2 fasting is consuming no more than 500–600 calories on two separate days each week.

Low-carbohydrate diets call for consuming fewer carbohydrates overall while consuming more protein and good fats. There are several types of low-carbohydrate diets, including the ketogenic diet and the Atkins diet.

According to research, type 2 diabetics may benefit from improved insulin sensitivity and glycemic control with both intermittent fasting and low-carbohydrate diets. It's crucial to remember that these methods might not be suitable for everyone and that they should be addressed with a healthcare professional before beginning.

Also, because both of these strategies may restrict the consumption of particular nutrients, it's critical to make sure that appropriate nourishment is being obtained. Working closely with a healthcare provider and a registered dietitian can help ensure that adequate nutrition is being obtained while following these approaches.

It's also critical to remember that these strategies do not

take the place of other components of diabetes treatment including exercise, medication administration, and routine blood glucose testing.

Emerging therapies for insulin resistance and diabetes.

A variety of cutting-edge medicines, such as bariatric surgery and treatments based on the gut flora, are among the emerging therapeutics for insulin resistance and diabetes.

Research indicates that altering the gut microbiota may be a promising strategy for treating insulin resistance and diabetes. The gut microbiome plays a critical role in the control of metabolism and energy balance. The use of prebiotics and probiotics, fecal microbiota transplantation (FMT), and bacteriophages are just a few of the methods being researched. These methods seek to alter the gut microbiome's makeup, perhaps lowering inflammation and improving glucose control.

A medical treatment called bariatric surgery is used to help people with extreme obesity lose weight. Gastric bypass, gastric sleeve, and adjustable gastric bands are just a few of the different types of bariatric surgery.

Significant weight loss brought

on by bariatric surgery can

enhance glycemic and insulin

sensitivity. In some

circumstances, type 2 diabetes

can potentially be cured

through bariatric surgery.

Gene therapy, stem cell

therapy, and islet cell

transplantation are some

further cutting-edge

treatments that are being

researched. These methods

seek to get diabetes patients' normal insulin production and glucose control back.

It is crucial to remember that these cutting-edge treatments for insulin resistance and diabetes are still in the research phase and have not yet gained widespread acceptance. However, they represent promising avenues for future treatment and may ultimately provide new and effective approaches to managing these conditions. As always, it is important for individuals with insulin resistance or diabetes to work closely with their healthcare providers to determine the most appropriate and effective treatment approach for their individual needs.

Chapter 6

Overcoming Common Challenges in Insulin Management

Dealing with "burnout" and plateaus in insulin resistance. For people with insulin resistance and diabetes, dealing with plateaus and "burnout" can be difficult. Burnout is a state of emotional tiredness and disengagement

Breaking the Insulin Resistance Cycle

from diabetes management responsibilities. Plateaus are times when blood sugar levels remain high despite following treatment guidelines.

Working together with your healthcare practitioner will help you manage insulin resistance plateaus by determining the underlying cause and modifying your treatment as necessary. This may entail alterations to medication schedules, dietary changes, or increases or decreases in physical activity levels. Furthermore crucial are regular blood glucose checks and awareness of hyperglycemia's warning signs and symptoms, such as increased thirst, frequent urination, and fatigue.

Dealing with "burnout" can be more challenging, as it can be difficult to maintain the motivation and energy required for diabetes management over time.

Seeking support from family and friends, joining a support group, or working with a mental health professional to address the emotional and psychological aspects of diabetes management are all strategies that may be beneficial. Setting achievable goals and focusing on enjoyable and rewarding self-care activities may also be beneficial.

Furthermore, it is critical to prioritize self-compassion and recognize that managing insulin resistance and diabetes can be difficult and requires ongoing effort. Celebrating small victories and focusing on progress rather than perfection can help to maintain motivation and reduce the risk of burnout. Finally, maintaining a positive attitude and focusing on the benefits of effective diabetes management, such as improved overall health and reduced risk of complications, can also help to sustain motivation over time.

Coping with hypoglycemia (low blood sugar) and hyperglycemia (high blood sugar)

In order to effectively manage insulin resistance and diabetes, one must learn to deal with hypo and hyperglycemia.

Having a strategy in place for managing low blood sugar episodes is essential for managing hypoglycemia. This could include taking fast-acting carbs, like glucose tablets or juice, to swiftly elevate blood sugar levels. Finding the source of hypoglycemia and taking precautions to stop further incidents are also crucial. The timing of meals and snacks, the dosage of medications, or the amount of physical exercise may all need to be changed.

Blood sugar levels must be constantly monitored and the course of treatment must be changed as necessary to manage hyperglycemia. Increasing physical activity levels, changing your diet, or altering your prescription dosages may all be necessary.

Recognizing the symptoms and indicators of hyperglycemia is crucial and as well as taking steps to prevent future occurrences. This may involve avoiding high-carbohydrate foods, staying well-hydrated, and engaging in regular physical activity. Also, it's crucial to collaborate closely with a healthcare professional to create a personalized plan for treating hypo and hyperglycemia.

This may entail routine blood sugar checks, check-ups to evaluate general health and spot any potential issues, and continued therapy modifications as necessary. With the right care, people with insulin resistance and diabetes can reduce their risk of hypo and hyperglycemia and keep their blood sugar levels under control.

Long-term glycemic control tactics and complications avoidance techniques

For people with insulin resistance and diabetes, maintaining long-term glycemic control and avoiding complications are key goals. Here are some tactics that could be useful:

Frequent monitoring: Tracking blood sugar levels regularly can help people spot patterns and modify their treatment plan as needed. This may involve using a continuous glucose monitoring (CGM) system, self-monitoring blood glucose (SMBG), or both.

Medication adherence: Adhering to medication regimens is important for achieving and maintaining optimal blood sugar control. Individuals should collaborate with their healthcare provider to ensure that they are taking their medications as prescribed and make any necessary adjustments.

Healthy eating: A diet low in saturated and trans- fats and high in whole grains, fruits, and vegetables can help manage blood sugar levels and lower the risk of complications.

Physical activity: Physical activity on a regular basis can help to improve insulin sensitivity and blood sugar control. Working with a healthcare provider to develop a safe and effective exercise plan is critical.

Tobacco and alcohol abstinence: Smoking and excessive alcohol consumption can raise the risk of complications associated with insulin resistance and diabetes. It is important to avoid tobacco use and limit alcohol consumption.

Regular check-ups: Regular check-ups with a healthcare provider can help individuals to identify and manage any potential complications associated with insulin resistance and diabetes.

Self-care activities such as stress management, adequate sleep, and relaxation techniques can help individuals maintain motivation and reduce the risk of "burnout" associated with diabetes management. Individuals with insulin resistance and diabetes can maintain long-term glycemic control and reduce the risk of complications by implementing these strategies.

Chapter 7

Tips and advice from diabetes educators and healthcare professionals

Diabetes educators and healthcare professionals can offer useful tips and advice to people suffering from insulin resistance and diabetes. Here are a couple of examples:

Collaborate with a healthcare team: Diabetes is a complex disease that must be managed collaboratively. Diabetics should collaborate with their healthcare team, which may include a doctor, nurse, dietitian, and diabetes educator.

Concentrate on small changes: Making drastic changes all at once can be exhausting and difficult to maintain. Instead, concentrate on making gradual changes to your diet and lifestyle. Begin by incorporating more vegetables into your meals, or go for a short walk after dinner.

Don't be too hard on yourself: managing diabetes is difficult, and blood sugar levels will be difficult to control at times. It's important not to berate yourself when this happens. Instead, concentrate on how you can get back on track.

Educate yourself: When it comes to diabetes management, knowledge is power. Take the time to learn about the condition, including the role of insulin, blood sugar monitoring, and dietary suggestions.

Self-care should be practiced: Diabetes management can be stressful, which is why self-care is essential. Meditation, exercise, and spending time with loved ones are examples of such activities.

Stay motivated: Diabetes management can be a lifelong journey, so staying motivated and focused on your goals is essential. Setting small goals for yourself, celebrating your successes, and seeking support from friends and family can all help.

By following these tips and advice from diabetes educators and healthcare professionals, individuals with insulin resistance and diabetes can take steps towards better management of their condition and improve overall health.

Chapter 8

Resources and Support for Insulin Management

Diabetes advocacy and support organizations

There are numerous diabetes advocacy, education, and support organizations and support groups. Here are a couple of examples:

ADA (American Diabetes Association): The American Diabetes Association (ADA) is a non-profit organization dedicated to the prevention and cure of diabetes, as well as the improvement of the lives of those affected by the disease. They provide diabetes resources and support, such as information about managing the condition, advocacy efforts, and research initiatives.

JDRF (Juvenile Diabetes Research Foundation): The JDRF is a non-profit organization that funds research to find a cure for type 1 diabetes and to improve people's lives. They provide assistance and resources to people with type 1 diabetes and their families, such as information on managing the condition and advocacy efforts, and fundraising initiatives.

Breaking the Insulin Resistance Cycle

Beyond Type1: Beyond Type1 is a non-profit organization dedicated to improving the lives of people living with type 1 diabetes through education, advocacy, and support. They provide a variety of resources and programs, such as online communities, educational materials, and fundraising campaigns.

Diabetes-Sisters: Diabetes-Sisters is a non-profit organization that provides diabetes support and education to women. They provide a wide range of resources and programs, such as online communities, support groups, and educational materials.

The Diabetic Online Community (DOC): The DOC is a network of diabetes-related online communities and social media groups. It gives people with diabetes a place to connect, share experiences, and offer support and encouragement to one another.

These organizations and support groups can be valuable resources for people with insulin resistance and diabetes, offering a range of services and programs to support their needs and help them live well with their condition.

Tips for working with healthcare providers and managing insurance and medication costs

Working with healthcare providers and managing insurance and medication costs can be difficult for people with diabetes. Here are some hints to make the process go more smoothly:

Find a healthcare team you can trust: Look for healthcare providers who have experience working with diabetes patients and with whom you feel comfortable discussing your concerns and questions.

Communicate openly with your healthcare team: Inform your healthcare providers about any difficulties you are having managing your diabetes. Be open and honest about your diet, exercise, and medication regimen. If you have any concerns or questions, consult with your healthcare team.

Understand your insurance coverage: Examine your insurance coverage to determine what is and is not covered. Understand co-payments, deductibles, and out-of-pocket expenses.

Research medication costs: Examine the prices of medications and supplies at various pharmacies and online resources. Inquire with your healthcare provider about cost-effective alternatives.

Apply for financial assistance programs: Many pharmaceutical companies provide patient assistance programs to those who are unable to pay for their medications. Check with your doctor or go online to see if you are eligible.

Maintain accurate records: Organize all of your medical bills, insurance statements, and receipts. It is critical to keep these records in case of disagreements or questions.

Self-advocacy: Be an advocate for your own health. Speak up and ask for clarification if you have any concerns or questions about your care.

Learn about your condition and your treatment options. By following these guidelines, you can help ensure that you are receiving the best possible care and managing your diabetes in the most cost-effective and efficient way possible.

CONCLUSION

Finally, insulin resistance is a complex metabolic condition affecting millions worldwide. It is a significant risk factor for a variety of chronic diseases, including type 2 diabetes, cardiovascular disease, and fatty liver disease. While genetics and age play a role in insulin resistance development, lifestyle factors such as poor diet and lack of exercise are significant contributors.

Fortunately, there is hope for those who struggle with insulin resistance. This condition can be managed and even reversed with the right approach. This book has given readers a thorough understanding of insulin resistance, including its causes, symptoms, and risk factors.

In addition, the book provided evidence-based strategies for managing insulin resistance, such as dietary and lifestyle changes, exercise, and medication. These strategies have been shown to improve insulin sensitivity, decrease inflammation, and even prevent or reverse the development of chronic diseases linked to insulin resistance.

Breaking the Insulin Resistance Cycle

A comprehensive approach that addresses all aspects of insulin resistance is essential for successful management. Those with insulin resistance can improve their health outcomes and quality of life by making lifestyle changes and seeking appropriate medical care.

www.ingramcontent.com/pod-product-compliance
Lightning Source LLC
Chambersburg PA
CBHW061617250726

48653CB00026B/1627